Acne Cure - Natural cures for acne:

How to cure acne using natural homemade remedies and treatments

By Dr Rebecca M. Townsend

Table of contents

The Acne Dilemma

Whichile being one of the most common skin problems in the world, most people still have trouble in handling this annoying problem. We've all probably experienced this at one point in life. These reddish spots on the skin that often come with oily and sebaceous discharges can sometimes leave scars that can last for days or weeks, even worse, it can leave scars that can last for months or even years in severe cases.

Acne vulgaris or "acne" for short, is an incredibly common skin condition that often result in painful outbursts on the skin which can leave scars that last for a long time. Acne is characterized by the proliferation of pimples, blackheads, whiteheads, and oily skin which result from the sebum clogging up the skin pores. The worse part of acne is that it primarily affects the areas of the skin which are exposed, most commonly the face, but it can also grow in the upper chest, back, and shoulder areas.

While the physical effects of acne seem to be minimal and easily manageable, the psychological effects that it brings are tremendous which may include development of low self-esteem, anxiety, and in some severe cases, depression. This tells us that even though acne is a common skin problem, it shouldn't be taken lightly and should be managed properly.

There are a number of treatment options for acne, ranging from topical ointments that you can apply directly on your skin up to tablets that help in the skin's healing process to allow the acne-affected areas to subside and recuperate. However, these medications are made from different chemicals that can have nasty side effects. The use of natural ingredients to treat acne has been around for many years. And since the ingredients are natural, you can easily get them and you won't have to worry about the different side effects that most drugs bring on top of relieving acne.

There are certainly a lot of natural remedies for acne that just makes it confusing to choose one. This eBook features the best natural remedies to help solve your acne problems and allows your skin to recover its healthy glow.

I would like to share with you the different natural remedies for acne including their benefits, how to make each remedy, how to apply each one correctly, and give you short success stories from people (my previous clients) that have used these remedies for themselves when it comes to treating their acne problems.

Chapter 1: Apple Cider Vinegar (ACV)

Considered as one of the most powerful natural remedies that help in treating acne, apple cider vinegar is easy to obtain and even easier to make in your own kitchen; while not something that's relatively new, apple cider vinegar or ACV has been utilized as a natural remedy for acne because of its reliability, efficiency, and effectiveness as a treatment option.

Apple cider vinegar's anti-bacterial properties play a huge role in treating acne. The proliferation of bacteria is one of the major risk factors in the development of acne and the acetic acid in vinegar acts on the bacteria to protect the skin from acne.

Aside from its anti-bacterial properties, apple cider vinegar is also known to turn alkaline, helping the skin balance out its pH levels so that it's harder for the bacteria to grow and thrive on the skin.

ACV also acts as an astringent and dries up excess oil on the skin just like commercial astringents and natural astringents (ex. lemon juice). And because of this drying action, a good thing to remember is that you should be careful not to apply too much apple cider vinegar on the skin since it can cause excessive drying – this leads to the sebaceous glands to overcompensate by producing more oil on the skin, leading to an outbreak of acne instead.

The Benefits of ACV

Apple cider vinegar is known as an anti-bacterial and acidic solution. It's considered as one of the most powerful natural remedies for acne and using it on the skin provides a number of benefits which include the following:

- Kills off bacteria on the skin and prevents further proliferation of bacteria.
- Makes the skin more resistant to acne.
- Clears out sebum that tend to clog up the pores of the skin.
- Helps in regulating the skin's sebum production to prevent clogging up of the skin's pores.
- Helps in reducing inflammation of the skin.
- Exfoliates the top layer of the skin.
- Reduces damage from free radicals with ACV's beta-carotene content.
- Promotes a healthier and smoother skin complexion.

Apple cider vinegar can also be ingested and carry other benefits. Aside from those benefits that focus on the skin and in treating acne, ACV also has other nutritional perks that come along when ingested. Some of these benefits include the following:

- Relieves indigestion.
- Helps in lowering blood sugar levels.
- Prevents constipation.

- Boosts the immune system function.
- Soothes sore throat.
- Helps in lowering cholesterol levels.
- Alleviates muscle cramps.

Making Your Own ACV Solution

After knowing its numerous benefits for the skin, you're probably thinking that it may be difficult to make the apple cider vinegar solution. However, the ACV solution is simple and very easy to make that you can do it in your own home or in your kitchen. Here are just a few steps on how to make your own ACV anti-acne solution.

1. Gather the ingredients that you'll need:
   250 mL of clean water.
   250 mL of apple cider vinegar (organic, unpasteurized, unfiltered).
   500 mL container for the ACV soltion.

2. Dilute the apple cider vinegar with water, starting with a 1:1 or 1:2 ratio in your container.

3. Your apple cider vinegar solution is now ready to be used.

4. If you DON'T experience skin irritation, you can decrease the water or increase the apple cider vinegar in your ACV solution.

5. If you DO experience skin irritation, make sure that you add more water to the solution to dilute the vinegar.

After use, you can store the remaining ACV solution

How to Apply the ACV Solution

After learning how to make your apple cider vinegar solution, it's about time to learn how to properly apply it on your skin. It's relatively easy and you won't have a hard time using it by yourself by following these simple steps:

1.   Cleanse your face with water and pat until dry. This will wash away the bulk of the dirt on your skin, allowing the ACV solution to be more effective in treating acne.

2.   Lightly dip a cotton ball into the ACV solution and apply a small amount on your skin. This is to test if you're skin is able to handle the acetic acid in the apple cider vinegar.

3.   Once you see that there's no skin irritation, apply the ACV solution by using a cotton ball dipped in the solution and applying it directly to the areas affected by acne.

4.   Be sure to avoid applying the ACV solution near the eyes since the vinegar can cause irritation.

5.   Leave the ACV solution on for about 10 minutes. Letting it sit overnight is even better since you won't have to worry about the smell of the vinegar when you sleep at night.

6.   Wash off your skin with water thereafter.

7.   If you feel like your skin is getting too dry after application of the ACV solution, you can also use a moisturizer or lotion after washing off the ACV solution.

Case Study for ACV

This is a short case study/success story coming from one of my clients, she had written about her experience in using apple cider vinegar in dealing with her acne problems:

"Acne was always a problem since puberty and during my time in middle school, high school, and through university. I had a face riddled with acne which led to my low self-esteem. I've tried a number of acne treatments like skin cleansers and ointments, but none of them worked for me."

"I was starting to lose hope in solving my acne problems, but then Dr. Townsend recommended apple cider vinegar. Of course, I was skeptical like most people since it was something that you could find from your kitchen, but seeing how a lot of people said it worked for them, I gave it a try."

"In just a couple of weeks, my skin was

smoother, the scars were fading, my pores got smaller, and the blemishes on my face had grown lesser thanks to using ACV. Using ACV is definitely something I personally recommend when it comes to treating acne."

Chapter 2: Papaya

Whether in its raw or ripe form, papaya has been a long-standing treatment for a number of skin conditions since time immemorial, dating back as far as the 14th Century. After being utilized as a natural remedy for skin problems, which include acne, for centuries, papaya has built a good reputation in the world in promoting healthier and smoother skin. Even today, papaya still continues to be one of the most reliable remedies against skin problems, serving as an active ingredient in skin products like soaps, lotions, and moisturizers.

Originating from South and Central America, papaya later found its way to Asia, Europe, and eventually North America. Today, papaya is exported worldwide, both as a delectable fruit and as an ingredient in a variety of cosmetics.

Papain, the enzyme found in papaya, is found to be responsible in reducing inflammation and promoting healthier skin. Aside from that, papaya also acts as an exfoliant to remove the dead cells of the skin and replaces them with newer and healthier skin cells. The powerful enzyme in papaya also helps in clearing out the pores which prevents acne from developing. If you also want whiter and smoother skin, another popular benefit coming from the use of papaya is whitening the skin.

The Benefits of Papaya

Papaya has been a well-known ingredient in skin products throughout centuries, acting as an anti-inflammatory and exfoliant which provides a number of benefits to the skin and helps in treating acne which include the following:

- Reduces inflammation through Vitamin A.
- Promotes softer and smoother skin with beta-carotene.
- Prevents the formation of pus on the skin.
- Cleans out pores and prevents outbreak of acne.
- Clears the skin from blemishes.
- Keeps the skin soft by retaining moisture.
- Protects the skin from harmful elements like pollution and heat.

Exfoliates the skin to remove dead skin cells and make room for newer and healthier cells.

It doesn't come as a surprise that papaya is considered to be one of the healthiest foods in the world. Papaya still has a lot of health benefits when eaten as a fruit. These nutritional benefits include the following:

- Rich in fiber which helps in digestion.
- Boosts the immune system function.
- Lowers the risk for heart disease.
- Promotes good eyesight.
- Protects against arthritis and other inflammatory conditions.
- Lowers the risk for cancer.

Making Your Own Papaya Mask

Papaya contains a lot of benefits, whether it be eaten as a fruit or applied on the skin to achieve a healthier and smoother complexion. Making your very own papaya mask formula is easy and simple to make which will only take you about a few minutes. Here are the steps on how you can make your own papaya mask:

1. Gather all the necessary ingredients:
   One papaya fruit.
   A small bowl.
   A spoon (or anything to scoop and mash the papaya).

2. Cut the papaya in half and start removing the seeds.

3. Using the spoon, scoop up the flesh of the papaya and put it in the bowl.
4. Mash up the papaya flesh well until it has a softer consistency.

5. Your papaya mask is now ready to be used.

6. You can store the left over papaya flesh in the fridge for future use.

How to Apply the Papaya Mask

Now that you know how to make your own papaya mask, it's about time to apply it. Here are just the steps on how to use your papaya mask to treat your acne problems:

1. Start by rinsing your face with water to wash off the dirt and dust on the skin, patting it dry thereafter. Apply the papaya on your face, particularly areas affected by acne, forming it into a mask.

2. Leave the papaya on your skin for at least 15 minutes. This will allow the enzymes in the papaya to seep into your skin.

3. Lastly, rinse off the papaya mask using warm water. Wash off until the stickiness of the papaya wears off.

4. If your skin gets too dry after using the papaya, you can use a moisturizer or lotion.

Case Study for Papaya

The following is a short case study/ success story of which one of my clients had written about her personal experience in using papaya to treat her acne problem:

"I was always conscious about my acne problem. By the time I got into high school, pimples started breaking out from out of nowhere. I lost my confidence and started to try various treatments for acne, but none of them worked. I've tried almost everything from the drugstore – lotions, exfoliants, soaps, facial scrubs – but nothing worked."

"Papaya wasn't new to me since there are a lot of products that use it. But when I heard about applying the fruit itself, I was cynical. But there was no harm in it, so I gave it a try."

"After a few weeks, my skin was free from acne and it was a lot smoother, softer, and it even got whiter. Of course, I was surprised of the shocking results. I never thought that using the fruit itself could solve my acne problems! Definitely a recommendation for acne problems."

Chapter 3: Baking Soda

Well-known as a crucial ingredient in the kitchen, particularly for baking, baking soda can also be used to treat acne. In fact, baking soda can create one of the safest and most inexpensive treatment options for acne. Unlike other natural remedies for acne, the use of baking soda has actually garnered a lot of positive response over the years because of its efficiency and effectiveness in fighting off acne.

Baking soda or *sodium bicarbonate* is an amphoteric substance that acts by alkalizing the skin, neutralizing the acidic pH wherein irritation can occur or it can increase pH acidity whenever the skin is too alkaline. When it comes to acne, this balancing property of baking soda relieves the inflammation and irritation that come along with the development of acne. Baking soda also has antiseptic property which is used to combat the bacteria that is one of the biggest factors in acne development.

Aside from its antiseptic and anti-inflammatory properties, baking soda can also help regulate the amount of oil the skin produces. In turn, development of acne from the clogging up of the pores by the excessive amount of oil in the skin is prevented. Baking soda acts as a mild exfoliant, removing the dead skin cells to make room for the newer and healthier skin cells to grow.

Benefits of Baking Soda

Being an inexpensive and easily obtainable ingredient in the kitchen, it's a wonder that baking soda can be used as a natural treatment option for acne. It exercises its effects on the skin by balancing out the pH ratio of the skin which contributes to the development of acne. Other benefits of baking soda to the skin include the following:

- Relieves inflammation around the areas of acne.
- Balances pH levels of the skin and prevents further acne breakouts.
- Has antibacterial properties that removes germs that can cause acne.
- Acts as a mild exfoliant to remove dead skin cells and make room for newer and healthier skin cells.
- Prevents clogging of pores that cause acne.
- Removes excessive oil that the skin produces.
- Relieves itchy sensation on the skin.

With its surprising action as a treatment for acne, baking soda is considered as a powerful yet inexpensive remedy. Aside from the benefits that it brings to the skin, baking soda also has a number of nutritional benefits whether used as an ingredient in food or through alternative methods which include the following:

- Balances pH in the body and lowers the risk of kidney problems.
- Helps in fighting off cancer by altering pH levels of cancer tumors.
- Used as a relief measure for heartburn, indigestion, and acid reflux.
- Also used as a treatment for other skin conditions like psoriasis.
- Serves as an active ingredient in toothpastes and helps in removing plaque.

Making Your Own Baking Soda Mask

One of the greatest advantage in using baking soda as a natural remedy for acne is that it's usually available around the kitchen and inexpensive to obtain. After knowing how baking soda works in treating acne, it's about time to know how to make your very own baking soda mask. Here are a few simple steps that you can follow to make your baking soda mask:

1. Gather all the ingredients that you need:

    Baking soda (2 to 8 tablespoons).
    Warm water.
    A small bowl.

2. Put about 2 tablespoons of baking soda into the bowl.

3. Add warm water until the mixture becomes firm enough so that it doesn't

easily break off, but still moist enough to be able to spread it on your skin.

4. If the mixture becomes too moist, you can add more baking soda. If it becomes too dry, you can add more water.

5. Your baking soda mask is now ready to be used.

6. Make sure that you don't mix anything aside from water in the baking soda since it can react to other chemicals.

7. Before applying the baking soda on your face, test first if your skin is too sensitive to the baking soda mixture.

Applying the Baking Soda Mask

Now that you know how to make the baking soda mixture, it's about time to apply it. Here are the steps in applying the baking soda mask on your skin to treat your acne problems:

1. Start by cleaning your face with warm water and pat it dry thereafter. This is to remove dirt and debris on the skin and to make sure that the baking soda can stick to your skin and it does not fall off.

2. Apply the baking soda mixture on your face, making sure that you keep it away from your eyes.

3. Let the baking soda mask stay on your face for at least 15 minutes.

4. After 15 minutes, wash off the baking soda mask using warm water and pat dry thereafter.

5. If your skin gets too dry after applying the baking soda mask, you can use a moisturizer right after to ensure that the pH in your skin is balanced.

6. To get the most out of the baking soda mask, it is best to use baking soda that comes fresh right out of the box. Using baking soda that has been left in the fridge for too long may already lose its effectiveness.

Case Study for Baking Soda

The following is a short case study/success story coming from one of my clients after she had written about her personal experience in using baking soda as a natural remedy for her acne problems:

"Acne had become a long-term problem of mine. I was often conscious about my pimples, leading me to lose some of my confidence. I've used different skin-care products from exfoliants to facial scrubs, but none of them worked for me."

"I looked for different natural remedies for acne, but using baking soda got my attention because of a recommendation from my GP Dr Townsend, it was inexpensive and easy to use. I hadn't heard of baking soda being used as a treatment for acne, but I decided to give it a try."

"And just after three weeks, my skin was free from acne! I was certainly surprised at the results because I never thought baking soda could solve my acne problem. Even now, I'm still using baking soda on my skin every week to make sure that acne doesn't breakout."

Chapter 4: Avocado

Known best as a delectable fruit that is used in a variety of desserts and dishes, avocado contains powerful antioxidants that help in treating acne and promote the health of the skin cells, as well as vitamins and minerals that also help in protecting the skin from acne and other factors that can damage the skin. Because of the number of benefits that avocado can bring, the fruit has been used in a number of cosmetics, particularly in facial masks that can help in soothing the skin and cleanse the pores.

Out of the several natural treatments for acne found in this book, avocado has garnered a special standing because of how versatile it is when it comes to creating a facial mask to treat acne. Avocado can either be used alone or combined with other ingredients such as honey, egg whites, and even oatmeal to help in relieving acne problems. Because of the number of vitamins and minerals contained within the avocado, a healthier and smoother skin can be achieved.

As of today, avocado facial masks are commercially available in the market if you want to get smoother, blemish-free skin. Even famous celebrities are also using avocado facial masks to get healthier skin. But now, be glad to know that your very own avocado facial mask is easy and inexpensive to make.

Benefits of Avocado

Because of the high vitamin and mineral content of avocado, on top of containing power antioxidants, it comes as no surprise that the fruit has been utilized as a primary ingredient in several brands of cosmetics. Here are just some of the benefits that avocado brings when it comes to the skin:

- Helps in fighting off free radicals through its antioxidant contents.
- Keeps the skin moist and well-hydrated.
- Helps in fading scars from acne.
- Revitalizes the skin, letting it have a youthful glow.
- Treats excessively flaky skin.
- Helps in strengthening the skin.

On top of the benefits that avocado has for the skin, it also contains several nutritional benefits which include the following:

- Loaded with several vitamins and minerals.
- Helps in fighting off cancer.
- Promotes a healthy digestive tract.
- Lowers cholesterol levels.
Promotes healthy eyesight.

How to Make Your Own Avocado Face Mask

Unlike other natural remedies for acne, avocado is quite versatile in its use. Not only can you use it as it is, but you can also use other ingredients together with avocado for added benefits. Here are the steps on how to make your own avocado face mask:

1. Gather the ingredients needed:
   An avocado.
   A small bowl.
   A spoon or fork (for mashing the avocado).

2. Slice the avocado in half and begin scraping the flesh into a bowl.

3. Mash the avocado until it becomes pasty.

4. Your avocado face mask is now ready to be used.

5. You can also use other ingredients to mix with the avocado like honey, oatmeal, and egg whites.

How to Apply the Avocado Face Mask

After making your avocado mixture, here are the simple steps on how to apply your avocado face mask to treat acne:

1. Wash your face and pat it dry thereafter.

2. Apply the avocado mask on your face. Make sure that you avoid applying the mixture too close to your eyes.

3. Leave the avocado face mask for about 15 minutes.

4. Wash the avocado off your face with warm water.

5. If your skin gets too dry after applying avocado, you can use a moisturizer.

Case Study for Avocado Face Mask

The following is a short case study/ success story coming from one of my clients after her experience using the avocado face mask to help treating her acne problems:

"Working as a teacher, I have to take care of my skin. But ever since I was in college, acne was a problem that comes and goes often. I have to stand in front of people on an everyday basis, so it's making me incredibly conscious how my acne stands out."

"I tried a lot of acne treatments – soaps, exfoliants, moisturizers – but none of them worked out for me. I've tried cosmetics that contain herbal ingredients, but it really didn't work for me."

"After being recommended avocado, by Dr Townsend, I decided to try it out for myself. Who would have thought that using the avocado could solve my acne problem? Not only that, my skin also got smoother and my pores feel more relaxed after applying. It's a must-try and I've even shared this with my friends and family."

Chapter 5: Lemon Juice

Another fruit coming into the mix, lemon can actually help in treating acne. The secret lies in the juice of the lemon which relieves inflammation and helps in fighting off bacteria that can cause acne. The yellow fruit contains several vitamins and minerals that help in treating acne, but the most notable one lies in the citric acid content of lemon. This acidic content of lemon serves as the astringent which helps the pores to close and lead blemishes to dry up, resolving acne problems.

Today, there are a lot of cosmetics that contain lemon juice or lemon extract as an ingredient like in facial masks, astringents, and facial scrubs. One of the main strengths of lemon juice is that it's one of the fastest acting natural remedies for acne. In some cases, the effects are almost immediate that you can see the results of the lemon juice treatment just a day after of using it.

Lemon juice increases the acidity of the skin, making it unfavorable for bacteria to proliferate since skin that's too alkaline can let bacteria grow. However, despite the positive effects of lemon juice on the skin, it should be noted that it's not for everyone. When you have a dark skin color, avoid using lemon juice to treat acne since darker skin contains *melanocytes* which lemon juice can stimulate and cause more skin pigments to appear.

Benefits of Lemon Juice

Citric acid in lemon juice is the primary component that relieves inflammation. It also contains a number of vitamins and minerals that help in soothing the skin, fighting off bacteria, and even acting as a natural astringent that dries up pimples and relieves acne. Here are the benefits in using lemon juice for the skin:

- Fights off bacteria that can cause acne.
- Helps in regulating excessive oil production of the skin.
- Relieves inflammation on the skin.
- Acts as an exfoliant and dries up blemishes.
- Helps in fading scars on the skin.

Aside from its positive effects on the skin, lemon is a rich source of Vitamin C and has a number of nutritional benefits that include the following:

- Helps in fighting off cancer.
- Promotes iron absorption.
- Strengthens the immune system.
- Decreases risk for diabetes.
- Helps in preventing asthma.
- Lowers the risk for stroke.

How to Make Your Own Lemon Juice Ointment

The most important step in using lemon juice as a treatment for acne is in its creation. This is because lemon juice is highly acidic and can irritate sensitive skin, especially when it comes in its undiluted form. Before you apply it, make sure that you test lemon juice on your skin. Here are the steps on how to make your own lemon juice ointment:

1. Gather the things that you'll need:
    One tbsp of freshly squeezed lemon juice.
    Tap water.
    A small bowl.

2. In a small bowl, dilute 1 tbsp of lemon juice in 1 tbsp of water. If you find the solution still too strong, you can add more water.

3. The lemon juice extract is now ready to be used.

How to Apply the Lemon Juice Ointment

After knowing how to make the lemon juice ointment, applying it correctly is also an essential factor so you don't accidentally cause any damage. Here are the steps on how to apply the lemon juice ointment to treat acne:

1. Wash your face with water and pat dry thereafter.

2. Dip the Q-tip or cotton ball in the lemon juice and lightly dab it on the areas where acne is present.

3. Leave the lemon juice ointment on the skin for at least 10 minutes, depending on the sensitivity of your skin.

4. Wash your face again with cool water.

5. If your skin gets too dry, you can apply a moisturizer after.

Case Study for Lemon Juice Ointment

The following is a short case study/success story from one of my clients after he had used lemon juice ointment to treat her acne problems:

"I've been fighting moderate to even severe acne breakouts since I was in high school."

"Of course, I ended up using different skin care products for my acne like exfoliants and facial scrubs, but none of them worked for me. Even after spending more than $100 for these products, there was still no satisfying result."

"I heard about lemon juice, but I was a bit skeptical at first since I heard it can be irritating to the skin. But since there were some people who had positive results in using it, I decided to try it out too. I had thought that it would be painful putting lemon juice on my skin, but after diluting it, it actually wasn't that bad."

"After one week, I was amazed how my skin was free from blemishes! I've continued using lemon juice for a month now and my skin looks really different from before!"

Chapter 6: Garlic

No, you're not about to fight vampires all of a sudden. The use of garlic to treat a number of health problems isn't anything new since it has been used as an active ingredient in medicine as a natural remedy to treat infections and lower blood pressure. While it can smell pungent, garlic can actually help in treating acne because of its ability to fight off bacteria.

Due to its antibacterial properties, garlic has been used as a natural remedy for acne that's easy and inexpensive to make. Aside from that, garlic also contains a lot of antioxidants that help in repelling damage from free radicals like pollution, smoke, and dust which can contribute to the development of acne.

The use of garlic is not for everyone though. It should be a given that garlic or its juice should never be used in its pure form since it can irritate your skin or even cause blisters, so be careful. Be sure to dilute the garlic in water or other solvents like rose water or aloe vera.

Benefits of Garlic

Garlic is a natural antibacterial which provides a way to fight off germs without having to experience the side effects that commercial antibacterial drugs have. But aside from its antibacterial properties, garlic also has a number of benefits to the skin which includes the following:

- Rich in antioxidants and prevents damage from free radicals.
- Fights off bacteria that can cause acne.
- Dries up excessive oil on the skin.
- Antiviral and antifungal.
- Prevents inflammation.

Aside from its benefits for the skin, garlic also has several nutritional benefits which include the following:

- Helps in lowering blood pressure.
- Boosts the immune system.
- Aids in weight loss.
- Treats fungal problems like Athlete's Foot.
- Lowers risk for heart diseases.

How to Make Your Own Garlic Spot

It's important that you properly dilute the garlic in water since it can irritate or even burn your skin. Here are the steps on how to make your own garlic spot to treat your acne problems:

1. Gather the ingredients needed:
   2 to 3 cloves of garlic.
   Water.
   A small bowl or container.

2. Crush the cloves of garlic to get the extract.

3. Add 1-2 tsp of water to the garlic and let it sit for at least 10 minutes.

4. Your garlic spot mixture is now ready to be used.

5. Before using the garlic spot, be sure to test if your skin can handle it. If that's the case, you can add more water to dilute the garlic extract

How to Apply the Garlic Spot

After knowing how it's made, it's time to know on how to correctly apply the garlic spot on your skin. Here are the steps on how you should apply the garlic mixture to treat your acne problems:

1. Wash your face with water and pat it dry thereafter.

2. Using a cotton pad or cotton ball, soak it in the water where the garlic or garlic extract was diluted in.

3. Lightly dab on the areas where acne is present.

4. Make sure that you avoid the areas around the eyes since garlic can be irritating or cause a burning sensation.

5. Let it sit on the skin for about 10 minutes.

6. If you're worried about the smell, you can let the garlic spot sit overnight provided that your skin can handle the garlic.

7. Wash off the garlic spot thereafter.

Case Study for Garlic Spot

The following is a short case study coming from one of my clients after her personal experience in using garlic to treat her acne problems:

"I've always had a bad case of acne. I've tried a lot of skin care products, but none of them worked for me."

"Dr Townsend recommended that I should use garlic to treat my acne, but instead of eating it, she said I should apply it on my face like an ointment. I didn't believe it at first, but she eventually convinced me to use it."

"The first time I used garlic on my skin, I felt a burning sensation on the skin that hurt quite a bit. It wasn't easy and I wasn't looking for fast results."

"After enduring the mild burning pain from the garlic, in just three days, my skin is almost free from acne. Of course I was shocked! Tolerating the pain was actually worth it and the results were not only fast, it was reliable as well."

Chapter 7: Tea Tree Oil

The use of tea tree oil to treat acne isn't something new. It's a natural remedy for a lot of health problems, but its most notable use is for a variety of skin conditions which includes acne. Coming in as clear to yellow in color, it should be remembered that tea tree oil should never be ingested and only be used topically.

Since oily skin can contribute to the blocking of pores and the development of acne, you may find it strange to use tea tree oil to treat acne in the first place. But even though tea tree oil is indeed a type of oil, it's still different from the oil that the skin produces. Tea tree oil unclogs pores and removes excess oil to treat acne and prevent further acne breakouts.

Aside from washing away the excess oil on the skin, tea tree oil has antibacterial properties that also help in preventing acne by fighting off germs that can potentially cause acne.

Benefits of Tea Tree Oil

Because of its numerous applications on different health conditions, the use of tea tree oil is widespread around the world. Here are just some of the benefits of tea tree oil when applied to the skin:

- Fights off bacteria that can cause acne.
- Removes excessive oil on the skin.
- Unclogs the pores.
- Prevents excessive drying of the skin.
- Removes dead skin cells to make room for newer skin cells.
- Relieves itchiness.

Aside from its benefits to the skin, tea tree oil can also be used in a variety of conditions. Other health benefits of using tea tree oil include the following:

- Reduces dandruff.
- Prevents lice infestation.
- Used in treating psoriasis and Athlete's Foot.
- Can be used as a natural deodorant.

How to Make Your Own Tea Tree Oil Mixture

Tea tree oil should never be ingested and it should never be used undiluted. Here are the steps on how to properly make the tea tree oil mixture:

1. Gather your ingredients:
   Tea tree oil (small bottle).
   Water.
   Aloe vera gel (optional).
   Face mask (optional).

2. In a small container, dilute the tea tree oil in water with a ratio of 1:9 respectively since tea tree oil can irritate the skin.

3. Your tea tree mixture is now ready to be applied.

4. If you find the mixture too irritating, you can add more water.

5. Another alternative you can do is mix a small amount of tea tree oil to some aloe vera gel or face mask to still get its benefits but prevent irritating your skin

How to Apply the Tea Tree Oil

Before you apply the tea tree oil, see if your skin can handle it. If you can, proceed to apply the tea tree oil after diluting it in water or mixing it with other skin care products. Here are a few steps on how to apply the tea tree oil mixture properly:

1. Wash your face with water and pat dry thereafter.

2. For tea tree oil diluted in water, dip a Q-tip or cotton swab and start applying it on the areas affected with acne.

3. Let the tea tree oil sit for a couple of hours or even overnight provided that your skin can handle the tea tree oil.

4. Wash it off with water thereafter.

5. You can also mix tea tree oil with face masks or aloe vera gel, leaving them on for a few minutes and washing off thereafter.

6. If your skin gets too dry, you can use a moisturizer after.

If you feel like your skin is mildly swelling after using the tea tree oil, it will eventually subside after a few hours.

Case Study for Tea Tree Oil

The following is a case study/ success story written by one of my clients who used tea tree oil firsthand in treating her acne problem:

"I've been worrying about my acne problems for quite a few years ever since I graduated from university. I've used facial scrubs, astringents, and even some of the natural treatments for acne, but nothing seemed to treat my acne problems."

"I'm actually quite familiar with tea tree oil and even my brother uses it for his dandruff problems. But when I heard tea tree oil could treat acne from Dr Townsend, I jumped on board and decided to try it out."

"Knowing it was irritating to the skin; I followed how to prepare it properly and diluted it in water. The tea tree oil stung a bit first, but maybe because it was my first time using it on my skin."

"Four weeks after, the pimples on my face were gone! I couldn't believe it either, but that was just the cure I was looking for."

Conclusion

Acne is a problem that can go away! Sure, there are hundreds of commercial brands of cosmetics and skin care products that are available in stores, but most of them prove to be expensive or end up having meager results in treating acne. Aside from that, it's also often that we hear about the terrible side effects of some of these skin care products that prove to be more of a liability than what they're worth.

But you don't have to limit yourself in using skin care products that you only see on TV or find in beauty shops. Extend your knowledge and be open to the variety of treatments when it comes to acne.

I hope that this eBook has helped you in finding the best among the various natural remedies that can treat pimples and solve your acne problems. These have been some of the remedies that I recommended to my clients and I hope that you can also achieve the same results they had!

Thank you

I would like to thank you personally for purchasing or downloading this eBook during its promotional free period.

I hope that I have guided and educated you about the most natural and inexpensive ways to cure acne. Some people believe in using products from drug stores though I am a firm believer that one of the seven natural cures I have written about should help you get rid of acne or reduce it!

It is important that you follow the instructions above and apply these in the correct way and in no time you will have clean and clear skin!

I would welcome you to provide me with some **feedback** so that I can further improve the many books I will release in future. I honestly love to keep writing for those who like my work.

Please leave some **feedback** and I hope I can educate and enrich your lives with future eBooks that I release!

Warm regards.

Dr R. M. Townsend

www.ingramcontent.com/pod-product-compliance
Lightning Source LLC
Chambersburg PA
CBHW071013180526
45168CB00003B/1404